Counseling From Within: The Microbiome Mental Health Connection

Staci Duvall, M.Ed., LPC, AADC

Published by Staci Duvall, M.Ed., LPC, AADC, 2019.

While every precaution has been taken in the preparation of this book, the publisher assumes no responsibility for errors or omissions, or for damages resulting from the use of the information contained herein.

COUNSELING FROM WITHIN: THE MICROBIOME MENTAL HEALTH CONNECTION

First edition. June 25, 2019.

Copyright © 2019 Staci Duvall, M.Ed., LPC, AADC.

ISBN: 979-8224062263

Written by Staci Duvall, M.Ed., LPC, AADC.

Table of Contents

Counseling From Within: The Microbiome Mental Health Connection

Chapter One: Varying Perspectives

HISTORICAL PERSPECTIVE

Mental illness has been present throughout history and there are multiple explanations as to why human behaviors have deviated from the social norms and beliefs of any given time period. In an attempt to try and understand, identify, destroy, or treat those suffering with such behaviors, many theories emerged and continue to recycle throughout the centuries. Supernatural theory labeled people as mad, insane, or possessed by a demonic spirit. The belief of possession, displeasing the gods, eclipses, curses, and sin as causation of abnormal behaviors led to practices of spiritual healing and trephination (drilling holes in skulls to relieve trapped evil spirits) as early as 6500 B.C.

Somatogenic theory, on the other hand, labeled abnormal behaviors as disturbances caused by physical functioning that resulted in brain damage or imbalances in the body/brain. This belief rejected superstition and religion to embrace medicinal practices.[i] The most notable work is the theory of the humors which is associated with Hippocrates (c. 460-357 B.C.) and describes four distinct personality types. Hippocrates is known as the "Father of Medicine." His contributions to medicine are still honored today by the Hippocratic Oath—first, do no harm. In humoral theory, personality was classified in distinct forms (epilepsy, mania, melancholia, and brain fever.)[2] Deficiencies or excesses of black or yellow bile, blood, or phlegm along with seasonal changes were believed to cause a person's body to become out of balance and create mental illness. This belief did not stigmatize mentally ill people and allowed their families to care for them at home. Ancient practices of bloodletting along with the use of mercury, sulfur, or salt were also used to alleviate suffering and bring forth balance within the body.

The English and European governments became involved in care for mentally ill individuals and began the practice of institutionalization in "asylums" during the 16th to 17th centuries. Humanitarian reform began in the 18th century due to the poor quality of treatment and practices in place at the asylums and helped reframe how the inmates were viewed –from prisoners to beloved family members.[ii]

Psychogenic theory focuses on trauma and stressors in life which create maladaptive cognition thus leading to distorted perceptions and maladaptive behaviors. Treatment focused on compassionate care and physical labor for those living in American asylums in early 19th Century. Psychoanalysis become a dominant form of psychogenic theory treatment in the first half of the 20th Century and opened the path to modern-day cognitive-behavioral, psychodynamic, and client-centered approaches to psychotherapy (a.k.a. talk therapy).

Throughout history accounts of mentally ill individuals being tortured, ignored, shackled, sent to the countryside for compassionate care, treated with nutritious food or essential oils, taken to local mineral baths, institutionalized, de-institutionalized, medicated with psychotropic drugs, given lobotomies against their will, or left out in the streets and alleyways after institutions were closed for inhumane practices. Just as theories and practices in medicine have advanced over time, so have theories and practices in Psychiatry. To learn more about a full history of psychiatric care, please visit: https://nobaproject.com/ modules/ history-of-mental-illness

My favorite words of wisdom from Hippocrates are: "Let your food be your medicine, and your medicine be your food." Perhaps we (in the west) have strayed too far away from this wisdom. There is a way to integrate best practices of eastern and western medicine while honoring wisdoms from the past. I use the words integrative, functional, complementary, and alternative interchangeably to describe a holistic model of mental health care to accomplish this union.

Current Perspective

Currently, we use the term "mental illness" as a term for people with emotional and behavioral needs (abnormal behavior, cognition, or emotions). Most of us rarely question this term or current treatment protocols aimed at reducing mental health symptoms. We may tend to believe that tremendous progress has occurred in the way we view and care for people with mental illnesses in comparison to past practices with current technological advances, research, and ethical standards. Will we soon recycle an old theory, combine theories, or create a new theory to direct care of those will mental illness?

What is mental health or mental illness? Are these two terms interchangeable? How are these "diseases" diagnosed? How do we assess and treat symptomology (labeled as a disease) by our current nomenclature? Does complete healing ever occur for those with a diagnosed mental health disorder?

In his 2013, Dr. Thomas Insel former director of the National Institute for Mental Health (NIMH) raised a great question about the "Bible" of mental health diagnosing (known as the Diagnostic and Statistical Manual (DSM), currently in its fifth edition) with the following statement:

> *The strength of each of the editions of DSM has been "reliability"—each edition has ensured that clinicians use the same terms in the same ways. The weakness is in its lack of*

Did psychiatry take the wrong turn when it chose to become a part of the western medical model to avoid being delegitimized during a time when homeopathy, naturopathy, and Freudian techniques were being questioned and the pharmaceutical industry was booming?

A common example of this wrong turn in our current treatment model is a client with anxiety being prescribed medications at the onset of treatment by medical doctor with no counseling or holistic care. Benzodiazepines (Benzos), used primarily to treat anxiety disorders and panic attacks, are recommended to be used for two to six weeks in conjunction with antidepressant medication.[iii] Benzos are used in the short term until the antidepressant gets to a therapeutic level. Benzos have quickly become one of the most addictive and abused prescription drugs in the U.S. People have taken this drug for decades despite high death and addiction rates. Why have we strayed so far away from Hippocrates' wisdom?

Are counselors allowed to recommend efficacious integrative treatment options (i.e., alternative, nutritional, spiritual, naturopathic, and homeopathic options) to discover and cure underlying causes of mental health symptoms in our current model? If a "DSM diagnosed disease" is curable without medication, should it be labeled as a condition or known as one of life's challenges? Is mental illness a disease, or is it a symptom based upon our lifestyles and environmental factors?

It appears that with the advent of the current medical/disease-based model of mental illness, most clients seeking services are being treated with one-size-fits-all pre-established protocols. In the following pages, we will search for underlying causes of current DSM-based mental health symptoms, discover the power of food and toxins in mental health, discuss the role of the microbiome, and learn about integrative treatment options for counseling clients from within.

Integrative Perspective

Integrative medicine is the practice of combining conventional medical treatments with non-conventional ("alternative" or "complementary") ones.[iv] The general term more commonly known in the field of counseling and psychiatry related to integrative care is Complementary and Alternative Medicine (CAM). Instant images of meditation, acupuncture, massage therapy, and the use of herbs are conjured-up when Eastern medicine is mentioned. While these are considered alternative practices in Western medicine, integrative care incorporates practices from both foundations of medicine along with naturopathy and homeopathy.

The levels of integrative care vary by specialties—medical, psychiatric, substance abuse, aging, chiropractic, and counseling. Holistic practitioners exist in various areas of medicine (including dentistry). Naturopathy and homeopathy specialists provide distinct care based upon principles of their practices. Naturopaths focus on multiple treatment option to treat the "whole person" (i.e., diet, supplements, and herbs). While homeopaths focus on a singular system of treatment by using natural substances.

Is it any wonder these terms are confusing to people seeking treatment? Shameless comments or name calling related to alternative practitioners, including quacks, quasi-medicine, non-proven treatments, harmful treatments, non-FDA approved, witch doctors, snake oil salesmen, and charlatans, are pretty scary. It is difficult to know if you are on the cusp of an innovative medical breakthrough or wasting your time, money, and health on a total whack job when you go outside of mainstream medicine's practices. Just look at all the deaths and disabilities attributed to medical interventions.

CAM therapies are well established in the world of counseling and psychiatry—some, more progressive, regions of the country are further advanced in this practice. A mixture of relaxation-based counseling techniques, nutritional counseling, spiritual guidance, acupuncture, exercise (Yoga), hypnosis, biofeedback, and meditation are favorite choices in CAM. For me, CAM falls short of being truly integrative - holistic care by failing to assimilate comprehensive lab results involving the microbiome (gut) and whole body systems to check for underlying medical issues which mimic mental health symptoms.

The reason for this shortfall is that counselors cannot perform medical lab tests or interpret lab results as part of their scope of practice. Therefore, a combination of functional medical board certified integrative physicians, neurologists, licensed professional counselors, and homeopathic and/or naturopathic practitioners are essential team members in truly integrative counseling. Some psychiatrists including Kelly Brogan, MD and Daniel Amen, MD (with his team) have heroically created models for providing genuine integrative mental health care in their renowned clinics.

> *"Beyond conventional psychiatric treatments, functional medicine manages other factors with profound effects on mental health. It explores a wide array of interventions that are customized according to the needs of the patient. In combination with pharmaceutical and/or surgical interventions, functional medicine incorporates therapeutic diet, detoxification programs, counseling, lifestyle change, stress management and nutritional supplementation as part of the treatment. The aim of this treatment is not only to relieve the symptoms but to cure the illness and improve the overall health of the patient."* [v]

I hope to help you find a balance between the two polar-opposite ends of medicine through an integrative (functional) care approach. When integrative medical specialists begin to talk, I quickly realize that what I thought about medical care is very limited. Key words used in functional medicine include: inflammation, oxidative stress, genomics, metabolomics, toxins, detoxification, brain fog, autoimmunity, chelation, heavy metals, parasites, leaky (permeable) gut, food sensitivities, allergies, hormones, organic acid levels, Celiac disease, thyroid levels, adrenal stress, micronutrient testing, GI functioning, and many others terms I cannot begin to explain or pronounce.

What keeps me engaged in new learnings is my quest to find the cause and cure for symptoms versus treating symptomology alone. Diet, overall wellness, and detoxification are essential elements of functional - integrative care in counseling. This allows me, as a counselor, and clients to actively participate in the process of change by implementing strategies which complement best practices during treatment.

Personal Counseling Perspective

I remember fondly learning about the single most important and predictive factor for client success—the client/counselor relationship. It is my duty to develop and nurture a healthy therapeutic relationship to move clients into the next stage of counseling—reduction of symptoms. When clients report success at this stage we need to honor and celebrate the effectiveness of a strong therapeutic relationship guided by counselor interventions and aided by external factors in the lives of clients (family, support, employment, faith, nutrition, etc.) versus medication management.

Some clients want to skip the entire process of relationship building and implementing interventions and head straight to medication(s). This is a client's right, but it is not therapeutic in nature; it is medicinal in nature. There is a third option which is the integration of counseling and medication management. Allow me to clarify that I am supportive of using effective psychotropic medication along with counseling to save lives and reduce suffering. I am not against medication as long as it benefits more than harms a person's level of overall wellness and functioning. There are times I initiate the medication referral for clients suffering with serious mental illness diagnoses.

For clients with a primary focus on medication, I carefully consider the potential consequence of referring someone for a medication evaluation—both positive and negative. What happens if a prescribed medication makes my client worse or they become sick from side effects? Have I damaged the client/counselor relationship? Have I been less than efficacious with treatment options, or reduced trust with my client? Clients deserve to know that prescription drugs usage often turns into a circular process of having to take additional medications to reduce unintentional side effects and may create substance misuse or dependency. The potential consequences of medication management makes closing counseling services more complicated as clients often leave services due to frustrations from negative side effects or a false sense of wellness from medication before services are complete.

Consider this, if I go see a doctor and report extreme foot pain, the doctor may prescribe pain killers to help me cope with the symptom–pain. If the doctor doesn't ask why my foot is hurting, examine my foot, or x-ray the bone, he is treating symptoms. If the doctor does not discover that I have a broken bone or hairline fracture in my foot, how will my foot ever fully heal? Will I remain on pain medication for years as I further damage my foot by not knowing the cause of my pain? As Dr. Insel pointed out in his earlier quote, western medicine uses objective laboratory measures – not symptomology alone for medical conditions.

Clients often seek counseling to learn healthy behaviors and coping skills, discuss their lives, develop boundaries in relationships, and to work through deeply hidden internal pain or conflict. They do not come to me for a prescription or for me to ignore the underlying problem which is causing their distress. They want me to help them discover the root of their problem(s). As a counselor, I do not write prescriptions. Clients who are willing to see me for multiple sessions over a set period of time, pay for services, and dedicate themselves to changing their thoughts, feelings, or behaviors have a strong desire to change.

If I focus entirely on diagnosing symptoms and medication management how will my clients recover or heal? Will they fail because the underlying culprit (much like the broken foot analogy) remains hidden? Can an unhealthy digestive system create symptoms of psychological distress which mimic diagnostic criteria of mental health conditions? How do food, lifestyle, exercise, and spirituality play a role in overall wellness?

I think about the connection between personal choices and subsequent behaviors. I know that I experience a profound change in my mood, behavior, and thoughts after having excessive amounts of caffeine, junk food, or sugar. I become physically sick, overly emotional, and irritable. Most of us have probably seen a kid become hyperactive and overly emotional after eating a bag of Cheetos and drinking twenty ounces of soda or red punch. Consider the overall health of a person with food insecurity or inadequate nutrition.

Proper nutrition and healthy lifestyle choices are essential to proactive mental health. It is possible to integrate these approaches during the counseling process while still honoring the counselor/client relationship. It allows the counselor to focus on interventions which heal the body from within, and guides clients towards successfully closing therapy services with healing. After all, the ultimate goal we are all trying to achieve during treatment is overall wellness, not symptom reduction.

A person's dignity and ideal image of living are things I take very seriously. I continue to search for answers to help my client's thrive versus survive. I hope my writings will help create a paradigm shift in mental health care by considering the impact of the microbiome and ways to restore health. I believe when we discover and treat underlying causes of mental health symptoms that people heal.

Years of academia (Master's level), state board approved licensure, clinical supervision, and providing thousands of direct client contact hours have allowed me to form a strong sense of my professional identity and theoretical perspective of counseling. As a licensed professional counselor, I am trained to use Western medicine's disease-based therapeutic model which includes the following stages of counseling: developing a relationship with clients, diagnosing, planning treatment goals, reducing symptoms, and closing services. If an anxious person decides to seek professional counseling, I will begin the therapeutic relationship by building rapport and trust while assessing the client's symptoms, severity, and duration of anxiety.

Making a diagnosis of clinical anxiety includes the client's personal history and self-report, my professional observations, and I may also administer an anxiety inventory. My clinical duties remain clear—determine which one of the anxiety-based disorders best fits the client's reported symptoms. In other words, I match symptoms to specific pre-determined mental health diagnostic criterion from the current edition of the DSM.

After making a thorough diagnosis, I then focus on developing a treatment plan. Clients work directly with me to develop reasonable and achievable treatment goals which are aimed at helping reduce symptom severity and/or change the client's behavior(s). The treatment stage is based upon research and empirical evidence—it is methodical and purpose-driven. This all sounds reasonable, ethical, and logical—and it is.

Treatment planning also involves counselor intervention and specific techniques which align with my theoretical perspective (s). While the focus remains on building the client-counselor relationship and working on goals, another option is often requested by clients to alleviate their mental health symptoms—a referral for medication management. When counseling is supported with medication management, research indicates a higher reduction in symptom severity versus using counseling alone. While symptom severity reduction is helpful for clients, is it success in treatment?

I wonder if symptom reduction (especially with medication management) is actual healing or simply a mask of wellness. I know that other dynamics in clients' lives may mimic anxiety or mental illnesses (i.e., diet, exercise, lifestyle, spiritual needs, and medical or digestive issues). While I assess for these additional factors during the counseling process, I find that many overlook or underestimate the cause and effect relationship. Digging deeper into all aspects of wellness is essential to move past symptom reduction and address underlying issues for long-term healing.

Five (5)-Rs Perspective

Hippocrates' statement that our food is our medicine descends from a much older view of the world and nature; the Bible. Old Testament books address food, illness, prayer, essential oils, fasting, resting, and natural and supernatural healing. Today we seem to have deviated drastically from these teachings. Instead of openly discussing and learning about the healing properties of food, we choose foods based upon convenience, taste, appearance, ease, cost, and human desire.

It is difficult to discuss the attributes of healthy biblical foods without an expert, major corporation, governmental agency, or conspiracy theorist convoluting the conversation. Most of us just give up when talking about details related to healthy food. It has been passively added to the things we are told to never discuss (politics, weight, age, religion, and, now, food).

Therefore, nutritional counseling is a good place to start the conversation about the 5-Rs of integrative care: Remove, Replace, Repopulate, Repair, and Rebalance. [vi]

> 1. <u>Remove</u>: Whatever is either in excess or is a suspected (or known) sensitivity or allergen. Sometimes this requires a bit of investigative work and mapping of symptoms to see if there are patterns. Food sensitivities are tricky because symptoms may occur hours or days after exposure.
>
> 2. <u>Replace</u>: Once the offending foods and lifestyle triggers are removed, work on replacing the factors necessary to optimize

digestive secretions - enzymatic activity. In this stage, look at repletion of vitamins, minerals and other nutrients as well.

3. <u>Repopulate</u>: Restoring the balance of good bacteria in your gut is absolutely crucial to overall health. This involves using probiotic foods, fiber-rich foods, and sometimes a supplement.

4. <u>Repair</u>: The gut lining can be severely compromised during periods of inflammation, stress and when exposed to allergens over time. Repairing the gut lining is needed to ensure proper absorption of nutrients. This involves eating foods rich in zinc, vitamins A, D and C and amino acids, particularly L-glutamine.

5. <u>Rebalance</u>: This is where lifestyle really comes into play. It is important to address the external stressors that may increase your sympathetic drive in the nervous system and reduce the parasympathetic drive. Practices like yoga, meditation, deep breathing, good sleep and other mindfulness-based practices may help restore hormone balance that will protect your gut and subsequently, your entire body.

Integrative psychiatry - counseling is emerging with a shared meaning to answer the question: "What is causing mental health symptoms?" As the integrative medical model continues to grow and create changes within our medical care system, we must learn how to implement protocols from the 5-R functional medicine approach in mental health care.

<u>Inflammatory Perspective</u>

Inflammation may begin from a single source or from multiple sources. Determining the source(s) which causes an inflamed gut (microbiome) is the first step in the 5-R recovery program. Let's review the bodily systems (which are pathways for mental health diagnoses) to locate the source(s) of inflammation. The Autonomic Nervous System (ANS) has three subsystems: Parasympathetic (PNS), Sympathetic (SNS), and Enteric (ENS). The ENS is connected to the microbiome via the vagus nerve which communicates with the Central Nervous System (CNS) through the PNS & SNS. In other words, this nerve connects all nervous systems.

The SNS is known as the fight, flight, or freeze system. The PNS has the opposite effect of the SNS—the PNS is known as the rest and digest system. It conserves energy, slows the heart rate, increases intestinal and gland activity, and relaxes sphincter muscles in the GI tract.[vii]

Neurons communicate with other parts of the body through neurotransmitters. Ninety percent of communication is from the gut (microbiome) to the brain, not the other way around. Mental health and mental illness is often depicted as being a problem with the brain's chemical messaging system (neurotransmitters). Ninety-five percent of Serotonin (a neurotransmitter) is located in the gut (bowels) and fifty-percent of Dopamine (another neurotransmitter) is located in the gut. The ENS and brain use over thirty neurotransmitters. Acetylcholine is the main neurotransmitter used by the vagus nerve which communicates with all nervous systems.

Anxiety is one of the most prevalent DSM diagnoses in the world effecting an estimated forty million Americans per year.[viii] Imagine what the body experiences physically when in an extended state of anxiety or panic. What happens to the adrenals if a person's SNS remains activated? Dr. Jill Carnahan states that adrenal fatigue symptoms include: mild depression or anxiety, multiple food and/or inhalant allergies, lethargy or lack of energy, increased effort to perform daily tasks, decreased ability to handle stress, dry and thin skin, low blood sugar, low body temperature, heart palpitations, unexplained hair loss, and alternating constipation and diarrhea. If we are treating anxiety instead of adrenal fatigue, will the client improve? This is when it helps to have a functional medicine specialist on board at the beginning of treatment to address these underlying conditions we cannot find in therapy.

When you feel anxious or nervous, you may get the sense of "having butterflies" in your stomach. When you panic, the SNS has been activated and the fight, flight, or freeze response tries to eliminate a perceived threat. The "mother" system (ANS) is activated to release the neurotransmitter norepinephrine from the adrenal glands. A complementary (CAM) approach used to reduce symptoms of anxiety and panic is to stimulate the vagus nerve through rhythmic breathing, cold water on the face, humming, or balancing the gut microbiome.

Another CAM approach to determine an underlying cause for anxiety symptoms is heavy metal screening. Mercury is a neurotoxin and it blocks Acetylcholine action—which is the main source of communication for the vagus nerve. Mercury is a naturally occurring element that is found in the air, water, and soil as well as bodies of water and fish.[ix] The Word Health Organization (WHO) lists mercury as one of the top ten chemicals of major public concern. Industrial exposure is also a common method of mercury entering the body. Cosmetics, pharmaceuticals, batteries, and dental fillings (amalgam) are other common sources of mercury.

What happens when the vagus nerve is inhibited by a neurotoxin? Do counselors or psychiatrists ask about mercury exposure or test for mercury levels when treating a patient with symptoms of anxiety and/or depression? When mercury is the culprit, are we removing it (a process known as chelation) or adding a pharmaceutical neurotransmitter intervention to reduce symptoms of anxiety and depression? The pharmaceutical intervention is not going to work properly if the neurotransmitter is being blocked or not working due to an unhealthy microbiome.

I like to say that if we treat anxiety with an antidepressant (Serotonin drug), we need to make sure it can be used (absorbed) by the body effectively. We have to consider if the precursors to Serotonin are defective (5HTP or L-Tryptophan), if bacteria has caused an imbalance in the production of Serotonin, and if the gut is healthy enough to absorb and communicate Serotonin through the vagus first. What if Serotonin is not the culprit? There are many other factors to consider from a CAM perspective to help each individual client.

Neurotoxins, infections, parasites, heavy metals, allergens, yeast, prescription drugs, vitamin or mineral deficiencies, food intolerances, dysbiosis, vaccine injuries, genetic disorders, thyroid disease, hormone imbalances, underlying medical conditions, trauma, diet, exercise, sugar, artificial sweeteners, Monosodium Glutamate (MSG), stress, toxins in the environment (chemicals, pesticides, herbicides, insecticides, and pollution), cosmetics and personal cleansing products, cleaners, GMOs, and other factors collectively and uniquely influence each person's physical and mental health. We can find what lies within our own bodily systems with proper lab test results – this is the single most important factor in healing (discover underlying culprits).

Microbiome Perspective

Drastic changes in food production started in the 1960s and continue today with genetically modified organisms (GMO). These are man-made seed changes which go against the very rule of Nature as being the provider for our food and medicine. Some changes are aimed at meeting global food demands. Mass production and cheaper food prices continue to be a necessity for survival of the ever-growing populations around the world. Food preservatives are used to keep foods shelf-stable while food additives and dyes are used to make foods look more appealing.

Chemically created compounds, such as artificial sweeteners and monosodium glutamate (MSG), are added to food by manufacturers and by some as a dietary choice. Chemicals sprayed on crops, food storage changes, grocery store friendly packaging, and fast-food chain restaurants add to the creation of new health-related issues in our food supply known as toxins. Toxins destroy our gut health—the microbiome.

Changes in wheat production yield a crop with far too much gluten protein, which is related to gluten intolerance and Celiac disease. Milk products are consumed at an all-time high. Casein, which is a protein in milk, is linked to serious health and behavioral effects. Gluten and casein intolerances mimic an opioid-type response in the brain. These food proteins can cause behavioral symptoms similar to Attention Deficit Hyperactivity Disorder (ADHD), anxiety, and Oppositional Defiant Disorder (ODD.) GMOs are being introduced to our food supply like never before.

Toxins are all around us. Our bodies are limited in the ability to detoxify all these chemicals naturally. Children are especially vulnerable to toxins due to their age, developing bodies, and limited choices of child-friendly healthy foods. Toxic reactions are linked to inflammation and damage within the microbiome.

When the gut is out of balance—the body, brain, and behavior are out of balance. Reflux and IBS may actually be symptoms of an inflamed or toxic gut. Symptoms are just that, symptoms. *What is the actual cause of the disease?* This question is one we are not used to having answered by doctors. I believe that is why we are so challenged by the fact that food can heal many of our illnesses—far better than medication can reduce the symptoms. We take prescriptions and believe that doctors have all the answers to our health care needs. In reality, most doctors don't understand advanced nutrition themselves.

The good news is there are treatments that heal the gut by identifying and removing toxins which created symptoms of illness and disease. Once symptoms improve, is the medical disorder in remission, debunked, or cured? Whatever we decide, I feel certain that we will face a lifelong battle of avoiding and uncovering new potential malefactors in our food supply. New chemically concocted toxins are added to our foods without our knowledge. We must join together, learn, and advocate for the removal of toxins in our food, water, and environment if we want to live toxic-free.

One place to start is by understanding how food may heal us—not kill us. To learn more about how toxins almost destroyed my son's life and how we were able to heal him by treating his microbiome, please read my first book: *How Do I Help My Child: A Mother's Mission.*

Nutritional Perspective

Nutrients play a critical role in our daily lives by affecting our mood, wellness, and behavior. The expression "You are what you eat" has great depth and truth. Our western lives are inundated with poor nutritional knowledge and false beliefs about healthy diet and lifestyle. Let's consider all the sick people in the United States of America today. Despite the tremendous amount of published research and historical knowledge we have related to nutrition, physical and mental health diagnoses are rampant. The number of people taking prescription medication(s) is staggering. Our people are sick and toxic foods are contributing to the rise of illnesses and diseases.

How did we get to this point and will we continue down this path of a disease-laden civilization? Do we want to be known as the generation of illness and arrogance which chooses a life of ease over our responsibility to care for future generations and our planet? Imagine past and future practices of food production and healthy living; what will be said of the choices we are making? Are there unintended consequences we are ignoring and will regret?

Does food affect our health and behavior? I often get irritated by this question and have to remind myself that personal knowledge related to the toxic and healing properties of food is unique to each of us. Diets are often influenced by variables of cultural heritage including financial resources, family - personal habits, religious beliefs, education, advertisements, and physical access (to name a few). We currently have numerous research articles, diet plans, cookbooks, and medical experts trying to explain how unhealthy food habits create diseases and lower our life expectancy rates. Perhaps there are too many competing views, convoluted plans, and commercial plans to choose from. This creates decision paralysis and avoidant behaviors due to cognitive dissonance (a term you will see me reference again which explains the resistance to new knowledge which does not align with one's perspective or personal knowledge).

Making food habits changes that are imbedded in our daily routine is a huge challenge—one which is often underestimated. I have never heard anyone argue that eating a healthy diet is harmful, yet I see few people able to sustain such. While we may each differ, we cannot continue to ignore the influx of psychological and physiological diseases plaguing our nation. We need to support one another and discover food truths which will unite us all and create a healthier narrative.

Counselors, psychiatrists, doctors, and occupational, speech, and physical therapists are inundated with referrals due to behavioral, mental health, and physical illnesses. Clinicians and physicians often prescribe therapies or medications for nutritionally-based concerns which essentially ignores the underlying cause of symptoms. Our disease-based logic is flawed. Instead of symptom-therapy-medication we need to switch to prevention-diagnostic lab results-healthy diet.

Based upon our current nomenclature, when kids are hyper, disruptive, or unfocused they must have Attention Deficit Hyperactivity Disorder (AD/HD.) An adult with stomach distress and gastrointestinal (GI) related illnesses must have Irritable Bowel Syndrome (IBS). A kid with indigestion after eating must have acid reflux. The defiant kids must have Oppositional Defiant Disorder (ODD) or an attachment disorder.

It seems like we randomly pick letters from a cup of alphabet soup to create a new label for everyday problems most of us may experience. Sadly, these letter combinations are well known to countless families today. Health care professionals may assume these labels are necessary or helpful to their patients as they provide answers and direct treatment goals. Doctors and clinicians want to make a proper diagnosis and develop individualized treatment plans to help patients succeed. So, why are so many people mired in the medical system for decades instead of thriving?

Instead, consider when a child misbehaves, gets sick, or displays symptoms of a diagnosable disease or disorder from a different lens. Did the symptoms begin shortly after the child ate a piece of pizza, chicken nuggets, spaghetti, grilled cheese, a sandwich, cereal, yogurt, cheese, or drank a cup of milk? Are these the only foods the child will eat? Does the child crave these foods? What is the normal diet of the adult seeking treatment for symptoms of irritability, fatigue, brain fog, and digestive distress? Are they nutritionally deficient or experiencing a food sensitivity reaction in the gut?

Could food be the culprit? "No way! *Right?*" Wrong! How does a food label create a human label? After ten years of research and experiences (both personal and professional), I have learned that food is most often the reason for unresolved labels (diagnoses) of chronic behavioral and medical health issues in kids and adults. If the foods are toxic, people are toxic.

When Western medicine cannot resolve or properly diagnose symptoms, functional medicine can often determine the underlying cause and provide healing with limited or no prescription medication. This paradigm shift focuses on the cause of illnesses (including any problem in our society), versus symptomology reduction.

Practical Perspective

Considering the debates related to diet, books, researchers, and the multibillion dollar food industry, I don't expect anyone to agree with everything I say when it comes to eating a balanced diet. One thing I have learned is that each person is unique and that individuality must be considered in every diet plan. For instance, after years of suffering from allergic and inflammatory reactions to different foods, I have specialized my own diet plan. I use research-based best practices along with biblical principles to help me nourish my body while avoiding complete misery from reactions to my food culprits.

I have to stay away from naturally occurring latex, nightshades, nitrates, sulfites, gluten, casein, and high glycemic index fruits. I avoid GMOs and limit carbohydrates to control my blood sugar and overall health. I have a background in teaching nutrition courses at the high school level. Nothing I learned or taught related to nutrition in academia or personal food allergy testing helped me determine the diet that works best for my body. Functional medicine's principles along with an elimination diet got me on the right track.

My son has a list of food sensitivities, allergic reactions, and toxic reactions to chemicals and naturally occurring benzoic acid. He must avoid preservatives, additives, GMOs, Aloe Vera, nickel, and many others. The fruits he can eat, I cannot (and vice-versa).

Whether I am grocery shopping, eating at a restaurant, attending an event, or stopping at the gas station for a quick snack, I am bombarded with unhealthy toxic food choices. Finding a healthy gluten, casein, toxic free (GF/CF/TF) food choice is like playing a game of *Where's Waldo* with an illustrator who uses my senses, brain, and innate desires against me. What to choose? What not to choose? Cravings, smells, subliminal and sublime messages on prepackaged junk food all work against my intellect and rationale until I either leave or breathe deeply and search for the things I can eat.

So, if I feel this way after ten years of living GF/CF/TF, I can only imagine what other folks think when I let them in on my secret love-hate relationship with food choices (especially living in the South). I write and speak about the challenges of living in a world where food is used as a weapon to harm our body, mind, and soul while giant corporations make millions (or billions) from their chemically concocted denatured addictive products they call "food."

Add in lies (oh, I should say well-researched non-biased information) from billionaire drug and medical companies who benefit from a population with chronic illnesses and psychological distress and it's no wonder why we are all confused about what to eat or not eat. In other words, it's not just me struggling with food choices. There are more "healthy" diet plans in today's society than you can count, much less name. One thing all these diet plan experts agree upon (except the dairy and wheat conglomerates and their allies) is that the American diet is horrific!

I have learned to refocus my anger and energy spent fighting the battle against corrupt food practices into simply making the best food choices for me and my family. I cannot fight these companies or make a reader follow suggestions and research-based best practices when it comes to food choices. Instead, I want to share my favorite foods. I know every nutrition expert will argue something against each of my choices and some folks will be allergic, intolerant, or avoidant to some of my food choices. No worries or judgement, these are my choices. There is no perfect diet plan since we each have unique needs, beliefs, and food preferences.

<u>My personalized diet plan includes the following</u>:

<u>Fresh foods</u> – those you find on the perimeter aisles of the grocery store (fresh fruits, fresh veggies), quality lean meats (fish, venison, chicken, and turkey), and flash-frozen fruits and veggies (if fresh is not an option).

<u>Quality oils</u> – extra virgin olive oil, coconut oil (saturated fat), and Earth Balance margarine spread (used sparingly).

<u>Rice & Quinoa</u> – (quality brands) including pastas and Asian noodles.

<u>Artisan GF flours</u> – Pamela's brand is my favorite for desserts and muffins (I also limit sugar).

<u>Restaurants</u> – yes, I eat out often. I love the memories, relationship building, and break from cooking or work. I make informed decisions and order off-menu items (separate choices the restaurant offers – like side dishes – in combinations that work for me). This has taken me years to perfect.

<u>Snacks</u> – these are important and are also very challenging. I eat plain potato chips (kettle cooked with oils of my choosing when I can find them) and snack bars from Enjoy Life or

Pamela's. Nuts, seeds, and dark chocolate are some more of my favorite snacks.

When we nourish our bodies with a variety of nutrition-dense foods, our health improves. I don't know anyone willing to argue against this common sense. Refocus your food choices and break the habits you have been tricked into or have become addicted to and you will see a difference in your body, mind, and spirit.

Chapter Two: Making Changes

———

"WE CHANGE OUR BEHAVIOR when the pain of staying the same becomes greater than the pain of changing. Consequences give us the pain that motivates us to change." - Dr. Henry Cloud, Christian self-help author

The Process of Change

It seems simple enough. *Change your food choices.* Healthy diet plans are everywhere; there are plenty to choose from. Most of us need to make changes in our diet, so why are we so resistant to changing our food habits?

Change is more difficult than most people recognize. Cognitive Behavioral Therapy (CBT) explains the stages of change as an upward spiral in which we learn from each stage as we relapse or fall back into old habits. We must identify where each person falls on the spectrum of change to really understand why someone seems unwilling to change. The Transtheoretical model stages of change include the following:

- Pre-contemplation - a person has no intention to change
- Contemplation - a person is aware a problem exists
- Preparation - a person is intent on taking action
- Action - a person's behavior is actively changed
- Maintenance - a person sustains change and new behavior replaces an old behavior
- Relapse - a person falls back into the old behavior

When we ask people to change their diet, we are not simply asking for them to change the way they cook or purchase groceries. We are asking people to change their lives. Food is an integral part of life. Our heritage is rooted in the foods we eat. Our lifestyles are based around the food choices we make. Whether we eat out at restaurants, prepare meals at home, stand in line at a local food pantry or soup kitchen, or miss a meal due to food insecurity, we base many of our daily decisions around food.

Diet plans ask us to change more than our food choices, they ask us to change our fast-paced American way of life. To embrace sustainable diet change, we must embrace that what many of us may know as healthy living is inaccurate. We must realize that we have been told lies about food and nutrition from the very experts we trusted. In other words, we cannot simply follow a new diet plan; we must learn why we need to change our diet/lifestyle.

Dr. Elisabeth Kubler-Ross explains the feelings associated with change have a positive and negative impact. As we face changes in our diet, we go from being a part of the "status-quo" to feeling like our lives have been totally disrupted. Shock and denial are feelings we experience as our "healthy" diet is being questioned. If we work through denial, we prepare to take action and change our behavior (diet). These changes are met with great anger and frustration.

While making significant life changes, we may get very angry and distance ourselves from new information (cognitive dissonance). Many of us get stuck in the negative impact of change. If we can make our way through the emotional roller coaster of being deprived of our normal diet and lives, it is possible for us to rebuild our lives through acceptance and commitment to lifelong change.

We must realize that our behaviors and emotions are impacted by outside influences - influences we may not be able to control. As we make change, we may be ridiculed by others. It is not our responsibility to change the world around us or the people in our lives. As we go through the stages of change and feel the positive effect in our lives, we must realize that each person has the power to choose. That power also allows someone to choose not to change.

So, how do we make change easier? First, we change by surrounding ourselves with knowledge, resources, and people willing to embrace change with us. Secondly, we must continue to read, ask questions, and seek the most up-to-date information related to diet and wellness. Thirdly, we need to share knowledge, develop skills, communicate effectively, and take time to learn new skills. Finally, we have to be patient as we adapt to a new way of interacting with food by allowing food to be consumed for optimal health.

Counselors are effective with encouraging and teaching clients how to create lasting change in their lives. We create goals, objectives, interventions, and use specialized counseling techniques. Counselors are natural change agents; we are trained to see alternative options and reframe automatic negative thoughts. Once we begin to understand the essential role of diet and nutrition in mental health care, we will be able to elicit lifelong healing and allow clients to remove the label of many mental health disorders. We need to work with our clients through dietary changes. There are some very creative ways to engage clients in the process of change.

Fables of Change

A fun way to learn how to create and sustain change is through a few fables including two mice and two men, a group of penguins, and two elephants. These fables depict situations where change is inevitable, yet scary. *Who Moved My Cheese?* written by Spencer Johnson speaks to people of all ages. Johnson tells the story of two mice and two men, all living in a maze where they must all search for food (cheese), which represents happiness and success. After living in contentment with an endless supply of cheese, they learn their cheese supplies will end soon.

Each character is forced to choose an alternative path to survive. His creative names for the mice – Sniff, Scurry, and the two men – Hem and Haw (which are based on human personality traits) allow people to identify and compare their own automatic thoughts and negative thinking patterns. The four characters are each required to create change on their own; go along with the change; resist change, change to survive; or continue to live in fear and die. This book makes you consider how you would survive if confronted with a major life change.

In their cleverly titled book, *Our Iceberg is Melting*, Dr. John Kotter and Holger Rathgeber illustrate the lives of a group of penguins forced to change when their iceberg begins to melt. Dr. Kotter is a world-renowned expert on change in the business world. He has written many books on the subject of change. His complex theory of change is simply presented when the community of penguins must find ways to save their entire population from catastrophic changes, which the penguins cannot control, that will destroy their iceberg. There are multiple relatable characters which correspond to humans handle change. Among them are thinkers, politicians, nay-sayers, gossips, leaders, and resisters of change.

Elephants are depicted in a poem by John Godfrey Saxe and a story written by Chip and Dan Heath. In "The Blind Men and the Elephant," Saxe describes how a group of six blind men visualize their vastly different experiences when encountering the same object – an elephant. Each man listed different characteristics of the elephant based upon the way he interacted with this massive animal. A wall, a fan, a rope, a spear, a snake, and a tree were each accurate interpretations of each man based upon the location he was in, yet they each failed to hear the description of the other men as they could not get past their own experiences (cognitive dissonance).

In the book *Switch: How to Change Things When Change is Hard*, authors Chip and Dan Heath use the analogy of an elephant and a rider. The rider, "the thinker," and the elephant, "the emotional energy," must learn to work together to initiate change. The rider needs direction, the elephant needs motivation (shared vision and common purpose), and the path (environment) must be clear and freed from obstacles along the way. They share how many different environments created and maintained substantial change. The rider must learn when to let go of things, how to rethink difficult issues, and how to get others involved who will help sustain change.

What each of these fables teaches us is that when we decide to make a change, we will encounter a vast number of people with different perspectives, feelings, and thoughts about what we are doing. That includes specialists, medical professionals, counselors, family members, and strangers. We will be asked what we are thinking and why we are doing these new things. We will feel like we are going crazy at times. Why is everyone against this change we are creating for our own wellness? Why do others get angry and shut down when we talk about our diet changes? Remember, as we go against what others know to be "the truth" and how they choose to live and eat, we face resistance and denial. If we are correct, others must decide to change as well or dismiss our thoughts. It is critical to know how others deal with change to help us stay on track and sustain changes in our lives and diets.

The Effects of Change – Ecological View

Efficacious counseling techniques provided by caring ethical counselors produce positive results in the lives of clients ready to make changes in their lives. Counseling teaches people how to set boundaries, cope with feelings, reduce negative behaviors, stop automatic negative thinking, process past experiences, reduce traumatic reactions, and stop addictive behaviors. It also provides numerous skills, and new techniques to improve overall functioning which reduces symptoms of diagnosable disorders. I cannot say enough positive things about the benefits of counseling in the lives of others.

People are not taught these things in school, life, or within family systems and they suffer for way too long by not seeking services. Counselors help people – that is the heart of what we do and why we come to work every day. We focus on the social, psychological, biological, environmental, and spiritual aspects of individual lives and how these factors influence the development of personality, moods, and substance-use.

What will future writers and historians say about the counseling techniques used during the twenty-first century? We are currently creating the history they will subsequently write. More importantly, how will those affected by mental health needs be treated in therapy? How long will people continue to suffer needlessly and take medications which create additional side-effects instead of healing a person from within?

Will people decide to make the changes we ask of them? Will junk food and processed "fake food products" win out over knowledge and logic? Are these things too radical and too difficult for the average person to implement? Will the pharmaceutical and big businesses win the fight due to money, power, corruption, and mind-altering substances? If they do, how will our medical system handle the influx of major medical diseases and severe mental health disorders? How will this impact our society, business sector, political system, and overall spirituality?

Bronfenbrenner's Ecological Systems Theory explores five levels of systems - environments which affects the development of a person: microsystem, mesosystem, exosystem, macrosystem, and chronosystem. We have to look at the way we are raising our children and how their futures will be shaped by our actions from each of these systems. To raise an overall healthy child, we must address their diet, mental health, microbiome, community, support systems, policies, family system, and faith (their culture).

The microsystem involves those immediately surrounding a child's life; family, friends, school or daycare, peer group, community, and faith members. Think about what a child eats, sees, experiences, and encounters from all these people. The interactions between these create the mesosystem. A child is affected by how he is treated by those involved in his life.

The exosystem involves greater connections which are not directly related to the child's immediate life - care (the parent's workplace and neighborhood). The macrosystem includes a distant collection of people and places that significantly impact the child's life. The child's view of life, cultural identity, beliefs, ideas, political, and spiritual views impact development (consider a child living in abuse, conflict, or a war zone) are included in the macrosystem.

The chronosystem involves the dimension of time and how long a child stays in a certain situation (living environment, family structure, divorce, parent's employment, and economic status during stages of development). These outside influences directly shape and influence the development of a child's life. The individual child is at the heart (center) of these external - environmental factors.

While many other theories exist to help us understand the developmental stages of children and how a person responds to events, biological predispositions, and psychodynamics of an individual, Brofenbrenner's theory helps explain how external factors in the environment of a person's life may directly impact overall development. Food, toxins, medications, political decisions, medical and allied health care (including counseling) practices, and cultural beliefs all impact a person's life and their overall wellness.

We must learn how to treat the whole person, not parts of the person presented to us in different levels of care. Collaborative medical, allied health, and mental health teams including: homeopathy, integrative - functional medicine, Ayurveda, complementary, alternative, dietetics, chiropractic, naturopathy, physical, occupational, and speech therapies, and Eastern practices (to name a few) must be formed at the local level and financially available to truly create and sustain a radical change in the way we view medical care in America.

Healthy foods, removal of harmful toxins, and open usage of quality supplements must become part of our educational system and lifestyles. We must disband the culture of fast and processed food products as a way of living – it is a way of slowly dying. Investing in the wellness of our own people must become a priority; not a luxury.

Complementary and Alternative Medicine (CAM) Changes

While researching integrative treatments to improve mental health symptoms, there are some themes which emerge: elimination diet, probiotics (including prebiotics), Omega-3s, Inositol, GABA, and the transmission of these via the vagus nerve. Using the connection of the gut-brain axis by adding probiotics and prebiotics which subsequently change the balance of bacteria to reduce mental health symptoms is an intervention known as psychobiotics.

Studies conducted from 2012 through 2017 have primarily focused on mice or rodents and the alleviation of anxiety, irritable bowel syndrome, depression, and gastrointestinal (GI) related disorders through the usage of psychobiotics via changing neurotransmitter communication via the vagus nerve. "Such findings offer the tantalizing possibility of using beneficial, or probiotic, bacteria to treat mood and anxiety disorders—either by administering beneficial microbes themselves or by developing drugs that mimic their metabolic functions. The new research also hints at new ways of managing chronic gastrointestinal (GI) disorders that are commonly accompanied by anxiety and depression, and that also appear to involve abnormal gut microbiota."[x]

"We're just scraping the surface," says McMaster University gastroenterologist Premysl Bercik, MD. "Definitely the animal data suggest that bacteria can have profound effects on behavior and brain biochemistry, probably through multiple pathways. Untangling those biological processes and learning how to apply that knowledge to boost human psychological health will take many years." While we await years of research, I beg the question, "What is it going to hurt if we use probiotics, prebiotics, and dietary changes to reduce symptoms of emotional and/or GI distress?" The usage of psychobiotics is a valid treatment option to use with clients as long as you know how to implement it. First, measure the effectiveness of symptom reduction by having clients chart subjective and objective changes. Have the client list symptoms, rate the severity of symptoms, and keep a written journal of changes in symptom severity while using each intervention. [x]

Secondly, the counselor will measure symptoms objectively with a screener or inventory (i.e., Burns anxiety scale or Beck depression inventory), note observed changes of symptoms with each intervention, and reassess with the same screener or inventory to provide evidence of improvement in symptom severity.

Thirdly, implement a complementary treatment plan. The following is an example of a complementary (CAM) treatment plan for anxiety:

Objective: Client will reduce symptoms of anxiety (i.e., restlessness, excessive worry, and irritability) from 8/10 on a Likert Scale to 6/10 by implementing the following: mood journaling, meditation, deep breathing exercises, massage therapy, exercise, psychobiotics (list types and amounts), and supplements (list types and amounts) AEB client's self-report, counselor's observation and Burn's anxiety score over the next 120 days.

Next, add Omega 3s while continuing probiotics. Lastly, add another intervention a few weeks later, and so on. Have clients journal the date of each intervention, supplement, improvements, and new symptoms or side-effects. If you wait sixty to ninety days to implement each supplement, clients will likely get frustrated or leave treatment due to financial or insurance related issues. Remember to have client change their diet simultaneously; otherwise, improvements may be minimal due to toxic or inflammatory foods being consumed daily.

Ask clients to seek an integrative medical specialist or medical physician knowledgeable with microbiome imbalances to begin the process of obtaining medical lab results to determine if parasites, yeast, toxins, heavy metals, or other imbalances are present. These need to be treated immediately and the client will need to involve the counselor with this process. The counselor may collaborate with the specialist/doctor with a signed release of information to help advocate and explain the severity of client's symptoms. The counselor may provide subjective and objective data (as explained above) which will help guide medical interventions. It always amazes me how much people will minimize their symptoms when a physician enters the room. They may open up to a counselor about issues they forget to report to a doctor. It has something to do with the white coat!

Start with the elimination diet to help each client identify which foods may be causing the underlying problem. If anxiety is being inflamed by gluten intolerance, the client needs to eliminate gluten first and rate symptom improvement. Probiotics and prebiotics are going to be essential throughout treatment to support the microbiome. The client may begin using these during the elimination diet. If the client alleviates symptoms with the diet and probiotics, there is no need for additional supplements (unless specified by an integrative specialist). Again, an integrative medicine specialist will provide lab work to determine if gluten or other foods are the real problems that require a needed change in clients' lives.

Diet Change

The University of Wisconsin School of Medicine and Public Health's Integrative Medicine Department of Family Medicine (UW Integrative Medicine) offers a six page elimination diet plan.[xi] The process takes a few weeks to over a month, depending upon the client's ability to stick with the plan and document all foods and drinks consumed during elimination diet. Typically, the foods someone consumes on a regular basis or craves daily are the culprits.

My son craved yogurt, cheese, milk, and wheat products. He was intolerant to casein (milk protein) and gluten (wheat protein plus other grains). When my son had his first integrative medicine appointment, his specialist immediately said to me, "You will need to get rid of his yogurt, cheese, and milk today." She told me that he was casein intolerant before getting his test results back, based upon her observation of what he ate during our three hour appointment.

UW Integrative Medicine proposes the following questions: What foods do you eat the most? What foods do you crave? What foods do you eat to "feel better"? What foods would you have trouble giving up? This is step one of their elimination process known as planning. During this first step, a daily food journal is shared with the medical specialist and/or counselor to help determine patterns of foods containing certain ingredients.

Step two involves eliminating all foods, snacks, and drinks which may include the ingredients identified as problematic. In order to determine which foods contain gluten, you will need an exhaustive list. These lists are available online or in books and magazines related to gluten-free living. Gluten-free Living[xii] has many helpful tips and resources available for free including recipes and substitutions. Step two is difficult for most people to complete as it is frustrating to read labels, realize how many foods include the ingredients you are avoiding, living without favorite foods, and having to write down everything consumed.

It is helpful to provide a handout to chart foods daily or to get clients to create their own food journal on paper, on their cell phone, or via a computer program (Excel spreadsheet). To make things more challenging, symptoms may actually increase during the first week of eliminating foods. If a client has gluten or casein intolerance, the addictive nature of these proteins can create a great deal of distress once intentionally eliminated. This is known as an opioid-type reaction to addictive foods. The good news is that once eliminated for a couple of weeks, symptoms should improve and the client should feel better. If not, have the client seek medical advice.

Step three involves challenging the system by reintroducing a food or ingredient, which once removed, made the client feel better. If the food causes symptoms to return or increases severity of symptoms, have the client stop using it again and see if you can confirm the initial results. Give it two days to see if the food creates problems again. If the client eliminates two or more foods at once, reintroduce one food at a time for two or three days and note any changes. Most people with gluten intolerance also have issues with casein and soy (a.k.a., the "trifecta"). Others may have cross-reactions to ingredients which the body may identify incorrectly as the offending ingredient. For instance, gluten cross-reactive foods include: coffee, yeast, oats, and dairy. Gluten-free oats also create issues for some people on a gluten-free diet.

Cross-contamination occurs when foods are crossed with others that include the offending ingredient. This may occur at restaurants, during food preparation, or while cooking. If a gluten-free food is cooked or prepared where a food containing gluten was cooked or prepared, cross-contamination occurs. This includes utensils, pots and pans, and countertops where gluten may have been present. Additives in foods and drinks may contain gluten and other "tricky" ingredients may also have gluten present.

So, if you feel like you have been exposed to gluten "a.k.a., being glutened" and experience symptoms of gluten sensitivity (i.e. bloating, headache, digestive issues, emotional changes, brain fog, or fatigue to list a few), you may have eaten a cross-contaminated food, your body may have experienced a cross-reactivity, or you may have unknowingly eaten a food containing "hidden" gluten. Don't give up, go back and look at all foods consumed, where you may have eaten at, and re-read food labels to try and uncover the source.

Step four (UV Integrative Medicine) includes creating a long lasting dietary change which I call a lifestyle change. Living without your favorite food and changing the way you interact with food is a lifestyle change, sometimes it seems radical and many others will challenge your new behaviors. It takes an unbelievable amount of self-control and sacrifice to change your food habits. Don't be surprised if you see clients slip back into old habits. Remember that the process of change includes relapse.

This is only one sample elimination diet available to use. There are countless others to help clients determine which foods may be creating symptoms of illness and emotional distress. While it may seem extreme, it is inexpensive to begin with an elimination diet and some clients will not have access to an integrative medicine specialist. If eliminating offending foods eliminates symptoms (or reduces symptoms), you have made a powerful difference in the life of a client. Giving clients tools to change their own lives is something they can use for a lifetime. Reducing symptoms with drugs is either temporary, masking of symptoms which continue to exist, or a lifelong prescription with long term side effects which may be worse than the original symptoms you were asked to treat in the first place.

For those clients wanting a simple fix with prescription drugs, work with them from the traditional medical model's approach while teaching them coping skills and using counseling techniques to help introduce integrative solutions at a later time (when the client has built rapport, reduced symptoms with medication, and has learned new skills). I call this an "exit strategy" from long term prescription drug usage. Some clients need to reduce symptoms with prescriptions in order to engage fully in therapy.

Change Strategies

Strategies are essential to help create and sustain diet - lifestyle changes for clients. The elimination diet is the first step to identify and remove inflammatory foods. To heal from within, we must add essential nutrients and healthy bacteria which balance the microbiome to try and repair or prevent damage. Next are some helpful global strategies to complement any treatment plan.

Strategy #1

Prebiotics and probiotics work together much like pre-cursors to Serotonin by aiding in adsorption and metabolism of Serotonin (which reduces negative side effects). Prebiotics team with probiotics to reduce symptoms of GI distress, inflammation, immune dysfunction, weight related issues, hormonal imbalances, and chronic diseases (including leaky-gut syndrome) by increasing the balance of good bacteria in the gut. According to Dr. Josh Axe, prebiotics foods include the following: acacia gum, raw dandelion greens, dandelion greens, leeks, jicama, under-ripe bananas, chicory root, garlic, onions, and asparagus.[xiii]

Probiotics are healthy bacteria which help your gut absorb nutrients and fend off infections ("build immunity"). This process begins at birth, in the birth canal itself and the mother's bacteria exposure to her newborn. A lack of probiotics creates a person with multiple illnesses including digestive, yeast, skin, and autoimmune disorders plus colds and flus (a sickly person). This person is usually treated with multiple antibiotics when they really need probiotics. Think about the irony here: treating a probiotic deficiency with antibiotics (which by definition destroy probiotics).

In order to absorb and metabolize probiotics, you need to avoid things known to destroy probiotics such as: antibiotics, tap water, sugar, genetically modified organisms (GMOs), grains, stress, chemicals, and certain medications.

The standard American diet (SAD) includes more sugary and salty foods than sour fermented foods. Probiotics live in sour fermented foods like kefir, sauerkraut, kimchi, coconut kefir, natto, yogurt, kvass, miso soup, kombucha, and raw cheese. Using ten to twelve different strands of active probiotics through supplementation will produce the highest benefit if you don't know what any of these sour foods are much less want to ingest them. Live cultures are better than dead cultures, live means refrigerated. Stability and potency of probiotics must be evaluated and researched to ensure you can actively use the probiotic purchased as a supplement. You need around fifty million CFUs (colony-forming units) daily. The different strands have complex scientific names, so try to find one with at least ten active strands listed on the label.[xiv]

STRATEGY #2

Omega-3s are polyunsaturated fatty acids found in certain foods containing Alpha-linolenic Acid (ALA), Eicosapentaenoic Acid (EPA), and Docasahexaenoic (DHA). ALA comes from chia seeds, green leafy vegetables, flaxseeds, and canola, walnut, and soybean oils (avoid rancid oils). EPA and DHA are found in oily fish, algae oil and krill oil. Americans often do not eat foods containing the proper amounts of Omega-3s on a daily basis. Dr. Axe recommends up to 4,000 milligrams per day for people with certain heart conditions, depression, anxiety, and cancer. Most agree that 250-500 milligrams per day of EPA and DHA combined will produce benefits. If you suffer with inflammatory conditions, learn more about warnings of Omega-6 which may increase inflammation over a period of time.

Omega-3s improve heart health, mental disorder and mental decline, reduce inflammation, fight autoimmune disorders, are associated with lower cancer risks, are supportive of joint and bone health, may improve sleep, benefit infant and childhood development, may reduce menstrual pain, are linked to lower macular degeneration, supports healthy skin and slows aging.

Mental health benefits seem to improve with Omega-3 supplementation. Some conditions being researched include: depression, anxiety, schizophrenia, ADHD, bipolar disorder, some personality related disorders, Alzheimer's, and age related decline.[xv] Barlean's Omega swirls are great quality and easy for children to swallow due to their smooth taste and flavors.

Strategy #3

Inositol is being studied to reduce the effects of depression, Obsessive Compulsive Disorder (OCD), Alzheimer's, insulin sensitivity, diabetic nerve pain, panic disorder, schizophrenia, ADHD, autism, psoriasis, polycystic ovarian syndrome (PCOS), high blood pressure, and metabolic syndrome. Whether it is classified as a B vitamin (B8) or a "vitamin-like compound," it is a sugar alcohol from rice bran and is found in many common foods. The best natural sources of Inositol include: cantaloupe, citrus fruits other than lemons, oats, beef heart, molasses, nuts, soy, bell peppers, tomatoes, green leafy vegetables, and bran.

Therapeutic dosage amounts depend upon the condition being treated, age, and other factors (six to eighteen grams per day is deemed effective for mental health symptoms). Negative side effects include: nausea, tiredness, headache, dizziness, and GI symptoms. From my experience, research, and training received from an integrative medicine specialist, Inositol may be highly effective in the treatment of OCD, ADHD, anxiety, and anxiety related disorders. The powder form is easy to administer to children and may be used two to three times per day with appropriate dosing.

Strategy #4

GABA (Gamma-aminobutyric acid) is a chemical neurotransmitter which sends messages between the brain and nervous system via the vagus nerve. This chemical is produced in the brain from glutamate. It may be used to treat anxiety (and related disorders), sleep disorders, mood issues, premenstrual syndrome, and ADHD. Gabapentin is a drug manufactured to mimic GABA and its effects on the brain. Low Serotonin levels and genetic factors may inhibit the efficiency of GABA receptors. This is not recommended for pregnant or nursing women, to be used in combination with other psychotropic drugs, or used in excessive amounts.

GABA is a non-essential amino acid combined with glutamic acid and vitamin B6. It has limited side effects, mainly sleepiness. Integrative medical specialist will help you determine effective dosage, genetic factors which may inhibit production and additional amino acids which affect GABA (Taurine, Glutamine, Theanine, and 5-HTP). Generally, up to 250-1,200 milligrams (split by two or three doses per day) are recommended to treat anxiety and ADHD symptoms. Start with the lowest dosage, work your way up (if necessary), and decrease dosage with any negative side effects. Valerian root, magnesium, and vitamin B6 also increase GABA levels naturally.

Continuing Change

Once we combine our knowledge of the history of psychiatry, modern day medical approaches, and functional - integrative medicine, we provide clients with options for their own care. Some clients want medication, period. Others will not do the work to change their diet. Some will slip back into past behaviors after seeing significant changes and making progress. While some will fall in the middle ground (partly compliant/partly non-compliant). I hope you remember that change is difficult and may be overwhelming at times.

Ayurvedic medicine is one of the oldest forms of natural healthcare. It stems from India thousands of years ago and promotes healing by using herbal compounds, diet, and other unique practices. Homeopathy began in 1796 and is based upon the belief that the body has the ability to heal itself by using "like substances" which create symptoms of illness (like cures like). Essential oils have the powerful ability to heal the body and balance moods. Acupuncture, physical therapy, chiropractic care, and exercise all provide additional healing for clients' symptoms of illnesses.

Detoxifying the body and skin are essential. This occurs through various means including: sweating, Epsom salt baths, saunas, exercising, fasting to rest organs, stimulating the liver to rid the body of toxins, refueling the body with nutrients, essential oils, activated charcoal, massage therapy, water, diet, sleep, coconut oil, and exfoliating. Learn more about how to take care of your body, mind, and spirit. The spirit heals in ways we will never be able to explain with science. There are numerous paths we may choose to follow which lead to complete healing.

Chapter Three: Practical Application – AD/HD

THERE ARE MANY OUTSTANDING practitioners pioneering changes with mental health care today. I think it is beneficial to see some examples of how a leading integrative specialist and brain-based specialist are implementing different treatment approaches to a common diagnosis of Attention Deficit/Hyperactivity Disorder (AD/HD). Many other common mental health diagnoses have protocols written by experts in functional medicine which you may implement with clients.

DSM-5 AD/HD Application

There are three sub-types of AD/HD in the current edition of the DSM which include: Predominately inattentive, predominately hyperactive/impulsive, or combined type. Inattentive types are often referred to as having Attention Deficit Disorder (ADD). Combined type meets criteria for both inattentive and hyperactive/impulsive. ADHD currently falls under the umbrella of neurodevelopmental disorders in DSM.

According to the American Psychiatric Association (APA), DSM-5's criteria for ADHD include the following[xvi]:

Predominately Inattentive type – six (or five for people over 17 years) of the following symptoms occur frequently (over the past six months):

- Doesn't pay close attention to details or makes careless mistakes in school or job tasks.
- Has problems staying focused on tasks or activities, such as

during lectures, conversations or long reading.

- Does not seem to listen when spoken to (i.e., seems to be elsewhere).
- Does not follow through on instructions and doesn't complete schoolwork, chores or job duties (may start tasks but quickly loses focus).
- Has problems organizing tasks and work (for instance, does not manage time well; has messy, disorganized work; misses deadlines).
- Avoids or dislikes tasks that require sustained mental effort, such as preparing reports and completing forms.
- Often loses things needed for tasks or daily life, such as school papers, books, keys, wallet, cell phone and eyeglasses.
- Is easily distracted.
- Forgets daily tasks, such as doing chores and running errands. Older teens and adults may forget to return phone calls, pay bills and keep appointments.

<u>Predominately Hyperactive/impulsive type</u> – six (or five for people over 17 years) of the following symptoms occur frequently (over the past six months):

- Fidgets with or taps hands or feet, or squirms in seat.
- Not able to stay seated (in classroom, workplace).
- Runs about or climbs where it is inappropriate.
- Unable to play or do leisure activities quietly.
- Always "on the go," as if driven by a motor.
- Talks too much.
- Blurts out an answer before a question has been finished (for instance may finish people's sentences, can't wait to speak in conversations).
- Has difficulty waiting his or her turn, such as while waiting in line.

- Interrupts or intrudes on others (for instance, cuts into conversations, games or activities, or starts using other people's things without permission). Older teens and adults may take over what others are doing.

There is no current lab test to diagnose ADHD. Diagnosis involves gathering information from parents, teachers and others, filling out checklists and having a medical evaluation (including vision and hearing screening) to rule out other medical problems. The symptoms are not the result of the person being defiant or hostile or unable to understand a task or instructions. [xvi]

Dr. Mark Hyman – AD/HD Functional Application

Dr. Mark Hyman (The UltraMind Solution) approaches ADHD from a functional approach by checking for additional symptoms related to inflammation, digestion, and nutritional deficiencies (to name a few). [xvii]

Dr. Hyman's Seven Strategies to Address ADHD and "Broken Brains" include the following:

1. Eat a real, whole foods diet. It should be free of additives, sugar, trans-fats[1], and processed foods. There is a close connection between the obesity epidemic we are seeing and the epidemic of ADHD and behavior problems in children.

1. Remove food sensitivities. While testing can reveal specific sensitivities, two big offenders are gluten and dairy. Partially digested dairy and wheat particles (called caseomorphins and

---

1. http://www.ncbi.nlm.nih.gov/pubmed/17181902

gliadomorphins) are found in the urine of severely depressed patients (as well as children with autism and ADHD). Dr. Hyman recommends a complete 100 percent elimination of all gluten[2] and dairy foods[3] for a full six weeks.

1. Address nutrient deficiencies. A host of nutrient deficiencies, including magnesium, zinc, selenium, tyrosine, and fatty acids, play significant roles in the development of ADHD. Many of these nutrients work synergistically. A Functional Medicine practitioner can custom-design a nutrient plan.

1. Fix your gut. Dr. Hyman has found the gut to be the source of inestimable suffering. He has found remarkable discoveries and cures that hold the promise of getting relief from common "functional" gastrointestinal symptoms (and most allergic and autoimmune diseases that originate in the gut), but also from everything from depression to autism, to OCD, to ADHD, to dementia and Parkinson's disease.

1. Eat an anti-inflammatory diet. Inflammation has been linked to almost all brain problems such as autism, ADHD, Alzheimer's, and depression. These and other diseases are all related to elevated levels of cytokines and systemic inflammation. They can cause problems in every organ[4], in every part of the body. Besides supplementing with fatty acids, you will want to eat an anti-inflammatory diet rich in wild-caught fish and plant foods like flaxseed.

1. Consume plenty of antioxidants. Oxidative stress[5] and

2. http://drhyman.com/blog/2011/03/17/gluten-what-you-dont-know-might-kill-you/

3. http://drhyman.com/blog/2010/06/24/dairy-6-reasons-you-should-avoid-it-at-all-costs-2/

4. http://www.ncbi.nlm.nih.gov/pubmed/16166805

5. http://drhyman.com/blog/2010/04/28/ultrawellness-lesson-6-energy-mitochondria-oxidative-

glutathione[6] deficiency have been connected to dementia, depression, Parkinson's, autism, and ADHD. An antioxidant-rich diet[7] includes plenty of colorful plant foods.

1. Detoxify. An overload of heavy metals in children who are genetically susceptible to their effects is one of the root causes of ADHD and broken brains. Each person responds differently to toxins. Some are great detoxifiers; others, like those with ADHD, are often not.

Dr. Daniel Amen – AD/HD Brain-Based Application: 7 Types

Dr. Daniel Amen (Amen Clinics) states that, "ADHD affects many areas of the brain–the prefrontal cortex and cerebellum primarily, but also the anterior cingulate, the temporal lobes, the basal ganglia, and the limbic system. The seven types of ADHD are based around three neurotransmitters—dopamine, Serotonin, and GABA." [xviii] [xix]

Type One: Classic

This first type of ADD is usually evident early in life. As babies, they tend to be colicky, active and wiggly. As children, they tend to be restless, noisy, talkative, impulsive and demanding. Their hyperactivity and conflict-driven behavior gets everyone's attention early on.

Common Symptoms in Classic ADD include: inattentive, easily distracted, disorganized, impulsive, poor follow through, trouble listening when others talk to them, making careless mistakes - poor

stress/

6. http://drhyman.com/blog/2010/05/12/what-is-glutathione-and-how-do-i-get-more-of-it/

7. http://drhyman.com/blog/tag/antioxidants/

attention to detail, forgetfulness, restlessness, being fidgety, difficulty awaiting their turn, act as though driven by a motor, being noisy, talking excessively, and interrupting others.

Dr. Amen uses scans of the brain called SPECT scans (Single-photon emission computed tomography) to determine blood flow volume through arteries and veins. This is an approach where integrative medicine is at its best; using alternative treatments to heal specific conditions with objective laboratory results.

Dr. Amen's treatment options for Classic ADD are aimed at boosting dopamine levels to increase focus. That is accomplished through either stimulate medications or stimulating supplements like rhodiola, green tea, ginseng, and the amino acid L-tyrosine. Getting lots of physical activity also helps increase dopamine along with taking fish oil supplements high in EPA and DHA.[xviii]

Type Two: Inattentive

Inattentive ADD is the second most common type of ADD. Those suffering with this type are usually quiet, more introverted and appear to daydream a lot. They may be labeled as unmotivated—even slow or lazy. Inattentive ADD is common but is often missed because children with this type tend to have fewer behavioral problems.

Common Symptoms in Inattentive ADD Include: trouble focusing, easily distracted, disorganized, poor follow through, trouble listening when others talk to them, problems with time management, tendency to lose things, making careless mistakes; poor attention to detail, forgetfulness, excessive daydreaming, complaints of being bored, appearing unmotivated or apathetic, being tired, sluggish or slow moving, and appearing "spacey" or preoccupied.

Dr. Amen's treatment options for Inattentive ADD are aimed at boosting dopamine levels. L-tyrosine (an amino acid which is the building block of dopamine), stimulate drugs, high-protein low-carbohydrate diet, and regular exercise are all treatment options.[xviii]

Type Three: Over-focused

In order to focus, it is necessary to continually be able to shift your attention. People suffering with Over-focused ADD have most of the ADD features, but rather than not being able to pay attention, they have difficulty shifting their attention; they become hyper-focused on certain things while tuning everything else out. These folks tend to get stuck or locked into negative thought patterns and behaviors. This type of ADD is often found in substance abusers as well as the children and grandchildren of alcoholics.

Common symptoms in Over-focused ADD include: core symptoms of ADD, excessive or senseless worrying, getting stuck in loops of negative thoughts, oppositional and argumentative, tendency toward compulsive behaviors, difficulty seeing options, excessive worrying, tendency to hold grudges, difficulty shifting attention from subject to subject, tendency to hold onto own opinion and not listen to others, needing to have things done a certain way or they get upset, and may or may not be hyperactive.

Dr. Amen's treatment options for Over-focused ADD are aimed at boosting Serotonin and dopamine levels in the brain. Treatment may be challenging as worry increases with stimulate drugs. Supplements are the first line of treatment including: L-tryptophan, 5-HTP, saffron, and inositol. Neurofeedback training and a low-protein diet along with some prescription medications (SSNRIs) are also helpful with this type of ADD.[xviii]

Type Four: Temporal Lobe

People with this type of ADD have the hallmark features of ADD plus symptoms associated with temporal lobe problems, such as issues with learning, memory, mood instability, aggression, temper outbursts, and sometimes, even violence. It is not unusual to see this type of ADD in people who have had head injuries.

Common symptoms in Temporal Lobe ADD include: core symptoms of ADD, memory problems, auditory processing issues, irritability, episodes of quick temper, periods of spaciness or confusion, periods of panic and/or fear for no reason, visual changes such as seeing shadows or objects changing shape, episodes of déjà vu, sensitivity or mild paranoia, headaches or abdominal pain of uncertain origin, history of head injury, dark thoughts (may involve suicidal or homicidal thoughts), possible learning disabilities, and may or may not be hyperactive.

Dr. Amen's treatment options for Temporal Lobe ADD are aimed at calming neuronal activity and inhibiting the over or erratic-firing of nerve cells. Magnesium is used to reduce anxiety and irritability. Anticonvulsants are prescribed to help stabilize mood. Learning and memory issues are treated with gingko or vinpocetine.[xviii]

Type Five: Limbic

In Limbic ADD, the prefrontal cortex is underactive during concentration while the deep limbic area—which sets your emotional tone, controlling how happy or sad you are—is overactive. Depression is also associated with over-activity in the deep limbic area, yet a person's developmental history in addition to some subtle differences on SPECT scans (between Limbic ADD and depression) helps us differentiate between the two conditions so we can choose the best course of treatment to resolve symptoms.

Common Symptoms in Limbic ADD include: core symptoms of ADD, moodiness, negativity, low energy, frequent irritability, tendency for social isolation, feelings of hopelessness, perceived helplessness, feelings of guilt, loss of interest in things, sleep changes (too much or too little), chronic low self-esteem, and may or may not be hyperactive

Dr. Amen's treatment options for Limbic ADD include: DL-phenylalanine (DLPA), L-tyrosine, and SAMe are supplements used. Wellbutrin is a prescription drug which is believed to increase dopamine. Imipramine is another prescription option. Exercise, fish oil, and diet changes are also treatment options.[xviii]

Type Six: Ring of Fire

In Ring of Fire ADD, there is a pattern of overall high activity in the brain. Those with this type tend to have difficulty "turning off" their brains and typically feel overwhelmed with thoughts and emotions. This type tends to do much worse on stimulant medications alone. Ring of Fire ADD can be related to some form of allergy, infection or inflammation[8] in the brain, or it can be related to bipolar disorder[9]. There are some subtle differences between Ring of Fire ADD and bipolar disorder in the scan data as well as some differences in the presentation of a person's symptoms. For instance, we have found that the kids with ADD tend to have their problems all of the time whereas bipolar kids tend to cycle with their mood and behavior problems. Adults with bipolar disorder have episodes of mania while adults with Ring of Fire ADD do not—their behavior issues tend to be consistent over long periods of time.

Of note: It is possible to have both conditions—in fact some research studies suggest that as many as 50% of those with bipolar disorder also have ADD. Common Symptoms in Ring of Fire ADD include: core symptoms of ADD, sensitivity to noise, light, clothes or touch, cyclic mood changes (highs and lows), inflexible rigid thinking, oppositional, demanding to

---

8. http://www.amenclinics.com/conditions/brain-toxicity-infection/

9. http://www.amenclinics.com/conditions/bipolar-disorder/

have their way, periods of mean, nasty or insensitive behavior, periods of increased talkativeness, unpredictable behavior, periods of increased impulsivity, grandiose or "larger than life" thinking, talks fast, racing thoughts, appears anxious or fearful, irritability, and may or may not be hyperactive.[xviii]

Dr. Amen's treatment options for Ring of Fire ADD begin with an elimination diet (to determine any food allergy or sensitivity). GABA and Serotonin are boosted with GABA, 5-HTP, and L-tyrosine supplements. Blood pressure lowering or anticonvulsant medications are also options for treatment.

Type Seven: Anxious ADD

With Anxious ADD, there is low activity in the prefrontal cortex while there is over-activity in the basal ganglia, which sets the body's "idle speed" and is related to anxiety. The ADD symptoms in people suffering with this type tend to be magnified by their anxiety. Treatment for people with Anxious ADD often includes both calming and stimulating the brain.

Common Symptoms in Anxious ADD include: core symptoms of ADD, frequently anxious or nervous, physical stress symptoms such as headaches, tendency to freeze in social situations, dislikes or gets excessively nervous speaking in public, predicts the worse, conflict avoidant, and fear of being judged.

Dr. Amen's treatment options for Anxious ADD are aimed at promoting relaxation and boosting GABA and dopamine levels. Calming supplements include: L-Theanine, relora, magnesium, and holy basil. Imipramine or desipramine and biofeedback training are used to lower anxiety.[xviii]

Final Thoughts

Having the knowledge that life brings us high levels of emotional pain, stress, toxins in our foods, and a drug for every symptom of distress, we must do our part as counselors to educate ourselves and our clients about natural ways to strengthen the microbiome and build immunity. Perhaps we need to learn more from past and current natural health practices. Living outside the current "norm" of acceptable medical practices is a must when that "norm" creates illness and lifelong dependency on pharmaceuticals and doctors.

I hope to challenge both counselors and clients to view their roles and treatment options from a new perspective. As a counselor, when a client comes into your office with mental health symptoms, which new techniques will you incorporate? As a client needing treatment, what will you now ask your counselor and doctor? I hope you will find solutions which heal underlying culprits of mental illness by *Counseling From Within*.

References

[i]Farreras, I. G. (2019). History of mental illness. R. Biswas-Diener & E. Diener (Eds), *Noba textbook series: Psychology.* Champaign, IL: DEF publishers. DOI: nobaproject.com[10]

[ii] Lagay, F. (2002). The legacy of humoral medicine. AMA Journal of Ethics. *Virtual Mentor.* Retrieved from https://journalofethics.ama-assn.org/article/legacy-humoral-medicine/2002-07

[iii] Anderson, L. Benzodiazepines: overview and use. Retrieved from https://www.drugs.com/article/benzodiazepines.html

[iv] American Psychiatric Association. Integrative medicine. Retrieved from https://www.psychiatry.org/psychiatrists/practice/professional-interests/integrative-medicine

[v] Dave, D. (2014). Functional medicine: can it you're your mental illness? *Integrative* Psychiatry. Retrieved from https://www.integrativepsychiatry.net/blog/functional-medicine-can-it-cure-your-mental-illness/

[vi] Boston Functional Nutrition. The 5 'R' approach to healing your gut. Retrieved from http://bostonfunctionalnutrition.com/the-5-r-approach-to-healing-your-gut/

[vii] Science Daily. Parasympathetic nervous system. Retrieved from https://www.sciencedaily.com/terms/parasympathetic_nervous_system.htm

---

10. https://www.nobaproject.com/

[viii] Anxiety and Depression Association of America. Facts and statistics. Retrieved from https://adaa.org/about-adaa/press-room/facts-statistics

[ix] World Health Organization. (2017). Mercury and health. Retrieved from https://www.who.int/news-room/fact-sheets/detail/mercury-and-health

[x] Carpenter, S. (2012). That gut feeling *Monitor on Psychology* (Vol 43, No. 8 page 50). Retrieved from https://www.apa.org/monitor/2012/09/gut-feeling

[xi] UW Integrative Medicine Department of Family Medicine. Elimination diet. *University of Wisconsin School of Medicine and Public Health*. Retrieved from https://integrativemedicine.arizona.edu/file/11270/handout_elimination_diet_patient.pdf

[xii] Gluten Free Living. Retrieved from https://www.glutenfreeliving.com/

[xiii] Levy. J. (2018). 7 reasons to get prebiotics in your diet plus the best source. *Dr. Axe Food is Medicine*. Retrieved from https://draxe.com/prebiotics/

[xiv] Axe, J. (2019). What are probiotics? A beginner's guide. *Dr. Axe Food is Medicine*. Retrieved from https://draxe.com/what-are-probiotics

[xv] Axe, J. (2019). Top 11 omega-3 benefits & how to get more omega-3 in your diet. *Dr. Axe Food is Medicine*. Retrieved from https://draxe.com/omega-3-benefits-plus-top-10-omega-3-foods-list/

[xvi] American Psychiatric Association. (2013). Diagnostic and statistical manual of mental disorders (5th ed.)

[xvii] Hyman. M. (2016). 7 strategies to address ADHD. *Dr. Hyman.* Retrieved from http://drhyman.com/blog/2015/10/21/7-strategies-adhd/

[xviii] Amen. D. Dr. Amen's 7 Types of Attention Deficit Disorder. *Additude Inside the ADHD Mind.* Retrieved from https://www.additudemag.com/slideshows/7-types-of-add-adhd-amen/

[xix] Amen. D. Types of ADHD Dr. Amen on healing the ADHD brain. *Additude Inside the ADHD Mind.* Retrieved from https://www.additudemag.com/slideshows/healing-adhd-doctor-amen-7-step-treatment-approach/

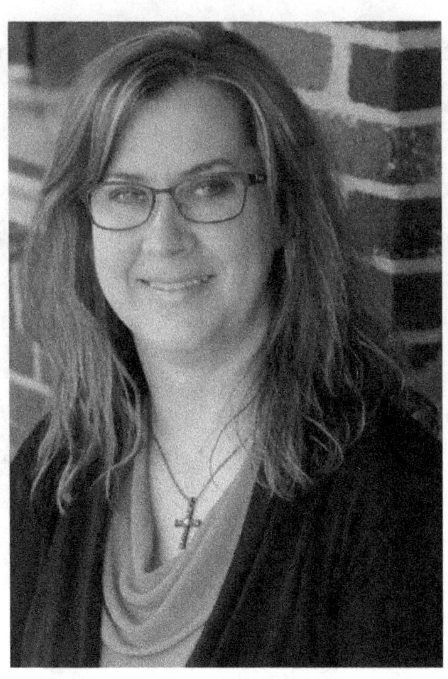

About the Author

Staci Duvall is a Licensed Professional Counselor with specializations in school counseling and substance-use disorders. She uses complementary and alternative methods which focus on microbiome health by using supplements, vitamins, and mindfulness techniques to help clients make changes from within. She enjoys helping children, teens, and adults reduce symptoms, discover potential underlying concerns, and find spiritual healing.

Staci earned her Master's degree from Arkansas Tech University as an educational leader in school counseling. She completed additional hours in community counseling at University of Central Arkansas and John Brown University. Her leadership experience includes serving on the board of Arkansas Mental Health Counselors' Association (ArMHCA) for three years, presenting at professional associations, colleges, and agencies, and publishing her first book in 2016, *How Do I Help My Child: A Mother's Mission*.

Staci's career experiences include teaching and school counseling in public schools, Director of Counseling and Disability Services at University of Arkansas Community College at Morrilton (UACCM), substance-use counseling at Quapaw House, Christ-centered private practice, and community mental health based counseling.

Staci's theoretical perspective incorporates Adlerian Therapy, Solution-Focused Cognitive Behavioral Therapy (CBT), Trauma-Focused CBT, Complementary and Alternative (CAM) therapy practices, and nutritional-based changes individualized for clients to discover underlying causes of mental health symptomology.

She is the proud of mother of two sons and has been married to Scott, her true love, for 26 years.

Read more at https://staciduvall.wordpress.com/.